Everything Changes with Brain Surgery

Bobby Simonds

Copyright © 2019 Bobby Simonds

All rights reserved. No part of this publication may be reproduced, distributed, or transmitted in any form or by any means, including photocopying, recording, or other electronic or mechanical methods, without the prior written permission of the publisher, and/or author, except in the case of brief quotations embodied in critical reviews and certain other noncommercial uses permitted by copyright law. For permission requests, email **bobby.simonds@gmail.com** . Serious inquiries only.

ISBN: 9781073559763

ISBN 13: **XXXXX**

Library of Congress Control Number: **XXXXX**

LCCN Imprint Name: **City and State**

Front Cover & Editing by author.

bobby.simonds@gmail.com

www.facebook.com/bobbyraysimonds

www.facebook.com/bobbyrsimonds

www.instagram.com/@bobbysimonds

#bobbyraysimonds

#bobbysimonds

#BOBBYRAYSIMONDS

#ATWISTINTRAVEL

#risenfromtheashes

#toxicamerica

#Challenge-thyself

#avoidinghavoc

#bobbyscreativephotographyseries

#QUESTIONINGREALITY

Books from Bobby Simonds:

1) A twist in travel: Fate (sci-fi)
2) The incident of 12/6/14 (nonfiction)
3) A twist in travel: Scientific Wastelands (sci-fi)
4) J.J.'s Rhymin' Adventures: The Complete Series (kid's poetry)
5) The True Masterminds of Manipulation: Volume 1 (nonfiction)
6) The True Masterminds of Manipulation: Volume 2 (nonfiction)
7) The True Masterminds of Manipulation: Volume 3 (nonfiction)
8) Living with Mild Cerebral Palsy (bio)
9) The true masterminds of manipulation: The complete series (nonfiction)
10) An angry memo: attention all humans (nonfiction)
11) Mind boggling experiences of the weird & strange (nonfiction/paranormal)
12) Missing my dog, my best friend: Ginger (nonfiction/self-help)
13) Don't mind the little things! (nonfiction/self-help)
14) Where are all the good drivers?

(nonfiction/self-help/educational)
15) Puggle fun with Ginger (picture book, young children)
16) Do you have what it takes to become the next great author? (nonfiction/self-help/guidance/educational)
17) Family in Ruins: The loss from a suicide (nonfiction/self-help/guidance)
18) What is banned in America: Volume 1 (nonfiction/awareness)
19) Risen from the Ashes: Untold Truths & Theories (Volume 1; Political Awareness/nonfiction)
20) Empty Conversations: Dear Dad (nonfiction/grievance)
21) Risen from the Ashes: You be the judge (volume 2; nonfiction/political awareness)
22) Risen from the Ashes: Surrounded by Stupid's (Volume 3; nonfiction/political awareness)
23) Risen from the Ashes: Living in an Unjust Society (Volume 4; nonfiction/political awareness)
24) A Twist in Travel: The End is Near (sci-fi/series)
25) Risen from the Ashes: Broken Shackles, Part 1 (Volume 5; nonfiction/political awareness)

26) Where are all the good drivers? Driving in Upstate New York (Volume 2; nonfiction/education/awareness)
27) Risen from the Ashes: Broken Shackles, Part 2 (Volume 6; nonfiction/political awareness)
28) Risen from the Ashes: Broken Shackles, Two-Fer (Volume 7; nonfiction/political awareness)
29) A Twist in Travel: The Final Journey (science fiction/action; volume 4; end of series)
30) Risen from the Ashes: Identity Crisis (nonfiction; volume 8)
31) Risen from the Ashes: The First 8 (nonfiction; volume 9)
32) Risen from the Ashes: Imprisoning America (nonfiction; volume 10, end)
33) Challenge thy-self: Phase 1 (nonfiction; philosophy, self-help; volume 1)
34) Challenge thy-self: Phase 2 (nonfiction; philosophy, self-help; volume 2)
35) Challenge thy-self: Phase 3 (nonfiction; philosophy, self-help; volume 3)
36) Challenge thy-self: The complete Set (nonfiction; philosophy, self-help; All three phases combined)
37) CNY: Customer Awareness (nonfiction; reviews)

38) Avoiding Havoc (single Novel, fiction; Suspense, Thriller, Action)
39) A Twist in Travel: The Complete Series (Sci-fi/Fantasy/Adventure/fiction/humor)
40) Toxic America: We Shall Obey! (Volume 1; nonfiction; self-awareness)
41) Toxic America: Concealing America (Volume 2; nonfiction; self-awareness)
42) Toxic America: The Conspiracy of They (Volume 3; nonfiction; self-awareness)
43) Bobby's Creative Photography Series: Volume 1 (nonfiction; photography)
44) Bobby's Creative Photography Series: Volume 2 (nonfiction; photography)
45) Bobby's Creative Photography Series: Volume 3 (nonfiction; photography)
46) Toxic America: The Perfect Simulation (Volume 4; nonfiction)
47) Toxic America: Broken Barriers (volume 5; nonfiction)
48) Toxic America: Crude Awakenings! (volume 6; nonfiction)
49) Toxic America: America's Emotional Distress (volume 7; nonfiction)
50) Toxic America: The Dome Effect (volume 8; nonfiction)

51) Hell has risen: Painstricken (volume 1; fiction; dark fantasy/thriller; suspense)
52) Toxic America: The Complete Series (Volumes 1-8; Nonfiction)
53) Questioning Reality: Volume 1(nonfiction; self-help; conspiracy; political)
54) Questioning Reality: Volume 2 (nonfiction; self-help; conspiracy; political awareness; conspiracy theory)
55) Questioning Reality: Volume 3 (nonfiction; self-help; conspiracy; political awareness; conspiracy theory)
56) Unfolding Misery: Pandora's Box (volume 1; fiction; drama, suspense, thriller, mystery)
57) Everything changes with Brain Surgery (nonfiction; self-help, inspiration, surgery, memoirs, spiritual, healing)
58) The Doctor's Call (fiction, series, mystery, thriller, suspense, fantasy, horror, mythical, legendary)
59) Unfolding Misery: Evil Matters (fiction, series, volume 2, drama, suspense, thriller, horror, mystery, dark fantasy)
60) Bobby's Creative Photography: Volume 4 (nonfiction; photography, spiritual, nature, landscapes)

61) The Real Jerry Lewis: Volume 1
(nonfiction; picture book, photography, pet's, family)

62) Questioning Reality: The first three
(nonfiction; conspiracy, self-help, political awareness)

63) Amazon's All-Star Self-Publishing Trade
(nonfiction; self-help, reference, guidance)

Chapter 1: The basics

Living life is full of challenges. Some good, some not. Whatever the changes, or the challenges we face – as human beings – we generally adapt; or deal with the nature of a new, unexpected path. It doesn't really matter what's thrown our way, we generally adjust.

Nevertheless, with having brain surgery, this hasn't seemed to be the case. I had undergone brain surgery in my Pituitary gland, back in the early summer of 2012. I had faced many challenges from this surgery. I was expecting to lose the almighty, hellish migraines, that I was having daily.

What I wasn't prepared for, nor was my wife, that my life had ultimately changed. The doctor didn't warn us about a personality change, or the permanent loss of memories. Some, various memories, had returned over time, but most have gone: deleted forever.

I didn't realize until recently – 2019 – of how much I have changed. I have a friend that is about to file for divorce. I will call him Tim.

Tim also had gone thru brain surgery in late 2017; and again, in early 2018. He too, has had a personality change – but not nearly as bad as I have. Like me, he has erased memories also. Which, when preparing for brain surgery, the doctor informs the patient with having a temporary loss of memory – not a permanent memory loss.

Tim, asked for his mother as soon as he awoke from his surgery. Unfortunately, Tim's mother not only died a few months prior, but he was there to say 'good-bye', and be at her funeral. Tim, has absolutely no memory of this ever occurring.

Furthermore, Tim took nearly a year to be able to return to work, with almost full working status. Unlike me, which took nearly 5 years, without the possibility of the doctor to back me up with fulltime disability benefits.

That's a lot of stress on my wife – that much, I realize. My taste with food has been pretty much the same; I barely remember what my father sounded like, or even what he looked like (perished in 2006). When I see pictures, I must stare at them for quite some time, for my brain to convey that the picture of him, was of course, my father.

One big issue that seriously has changed, is that I don't show affection, nor do I enjoy hugging; and I can hardly stand being, touched. It's something that occurred during my recovery; which in turn, is extremely difficult for my wife. Even my lobedo was supposed to improve, but only has depleted, almost altogether.

One great thing about the surgery, I did not have return, were those terrible migraines. I still get the occasional migraine, which is generally self-induced by stress, tension, or working (away from my writing; although if I write after 7 p.m., it causes headaches).

Working with the rest of the worker bees, has been the biggest challenge. I wasn't ever good with committing to a career (aside from being an author). But I was able to keeping a job from time to time. From October 2006 to 2008, a local McDonald's employed me. The following job was at a local factory, which I was employed (minus 8 months for a Recession Lay-off), was from 2008 until

2011. If it weren't for a few on-the-job injuries, I'd most likely still be there.

The following year, 2012, I had knee surgery, following with my brain surgery, only 8 weeks later. It was brutal, to say the least, as one believes they can imagine; they really cannot, unless you [or them], experiences it yourself [themselves].

I am just as stubborn as before, but from what everyone around me expresses (as much as they do), I may be more stubborn. Back to my lobedo; it is almost as though; my body believes my sex drive is on permanent retirement – which is difficult being in your 30s; whether I'm married (or if I were single). It is an intricate disregard, for the other partner. One can only come up with so many various excuses, before that person, concludes that it's related to the surgery. When, the person who had the surgery, feels as though it's gotta be something else. Either way, it makes you feel less than dog poo, when you cannot keep an erection, as a man. It angers you, rather than depresses you.

I used to be a rational human being. Now, I think I lost my way with rationality. And when I don't want to partake with something, watch out, that's for certain. My temper wasn't bad the first couple of years after the surgery. Nonetheless, with all the retraining, and loss memories, and confusion, it's no wonder why I have a temper, and others too.

If I were a vampire, I could relate. It's almost as though that my emotions have been, heightened. I know for fact, that I have a zero-patience level, and I am easily frustrated with myself and others, instantaneously.

Chapter 2: Signs

In my teenage years, I can speak from absolute memory, that I had depression. I recall my wife helping me thru it, before we became a married couple.

I know I don't have depression; I have frustration. I'm full of anger nearly all the time, because I'm forced to not be my old self – which I would prefer for others. But at the same time, change isn't always bad.

I met Tim 2 years ago. Therefore, I knew him before he had emergency brain surgery. He was in a car accident, which led him to surgery.

Unlike Tim, I had a brain cyst. Which I believe I received from the use of narcotics in my early, to mid-twenties.

I became a lab-rat for the doctors' in sunny, California. Thousands of dollars literally had gone for co-payments, and they wouldn't operate. It took nearly a decade to perform the surgery, and a different state. To say the least, I can tell you that doctors' care about the money: not the *patient*.

With all the specialists, and normal doctors' that I did have in Orange County, California, they were not in it for the patient. They claim, *"for the love of medicine"*, for the reason why they do what they do. Nonetheless, in our reality, ***"for the love of money"***.

I had one neurologist that literally prescribed me the wrong medication for anxiety (for panic attacks), that I had during the early stages; and I received anti-seizure medication – which hey, guess what? They caused seizures, and I lost the privilege of having my drivers' license – up until I had the surgery.

There were a ton of mistakes, and wrong diagnosis that I had received in California. Therefore, don't go and think that because you reside in California, that they have the best doctors. Doctor's are doctors. And one thing I've learned about doctors, is they're like cops, it's difficult to find the one that gives a crap about the patient/civilian. Another thing I've learned about doctors, is that they get a commission bonus from prescribing medication. Therefore, no matter what you suggest (for the medication), they only give out medication that they receive money, to hand out.

On an emotional level, however, I am like a bi-polar patient. My mood swings range from high to low, just like my energy. The difficult thing for me, however, is that for a few years, I didn't connect it with brain surgery, recovery. I assumed it was in relations with my Mild Cerebral Palsy.

Thanks to Google, you can locate nearly anything. But what Google doesn't list, is what patients may experience. It goes based on statistics, and what the medical field provides. Therefore, when doing research; look for blogs, or Youtube channels from real people, not those fakes, that want to rob you of your money!

A quick example, based with book searches, in relations to brain surgery. If you go onto Amazon.com and type in 'brain surgery' under the 'books department'; 2000 books listed. However, the first 10 pages that I scrolled through, only had one book, written by a real patient, ***"I had brain surgery, what's your excuse"***. Of course, the author had a few different versions, so it shows up a few various times through the ten pages I scrolled thru.

Nevertheless, out of the '2000' listed, a rough conclusion of 99% of the books provided are medical based. Hospitals, doctors, colleges, and so forth, were hogging up all the books, with an overpriced book price, no less. Majority of their books were for kindle price, $9.99 up $300.

You know majority of the kindles, that are published, traditionally, range around $10; thus, when I see a mark-up of nearly $300, you realize right away, that it's for school [or a professional field] – both of which, are an over-priced expense.

I get so frustrated with my current reality, that I enflame myself with my writing.

I don't read much, because I cannot focus. Majority of new authors (not all, but a lot more these days), are in it for the money. I am in it for the inspiration, the life tour, and the *escape goat*. The money would be great, the fame would be marvelous, but it isn't why I commit to *writing to the world*, as much as I can.

No, no, I'm here to inform you. Inform you with my own theories, hypothesis, experiences, memoirs, biographies (my own), my fantasies (my fiction works), and even my personal drama.

Unlike most authors, they don't reveal much about themselves, for majority of their books, that is. They leave cookie crumbs. I leave the whole cookie. I do this to let you know, you aren't alone with the way you think, feel, or experience something, that others may find outlandish.

I, myself, have been known to be outlandish with my theories, my UFO experiences, alien encounters (and other types of encounters), and even with my personal life. But like you, I'm still a human being (I hope)!

My wife and I haven't been "clicking" for some time. She is sex-deprived, along with a trail of financial hell. I cannot satisfy either ordeal.

Even when it comes to house-chores, I cannot keep up. Writing is my everything; even playing video games a few hours a day, is also my everything, followed with my pets! Without them, I would be completely hostile, along with if I couldn't smoke cigarettes.

You may be questioning why I titled this chapter: *Signs*.

The *signs* that I receive aren't about creating this book (or others), playing video games, or sharing my feelings. No. The *signs* are from my life, changing, the little things to the big. The drastically changing circumstances, that I feel I must jot down, encase you are mentally preparing yourself for brain surgery, or have someone close to you, that is brave enough, like me, who believes it will change their life for the better. It is significant for you, to second guess the operation. Unless you want a mid-life crisis to last until the day you die (or them).

Chapter 3: Mid-Life Crisis – Long Term

Experiencing a mid-life crisis is hell for the other person you are with, or those left in your family. But when it's lasting for, what seems like an eternity, from having brain surgery…. Well that's the eternal hell that your surgeon has brought upon you, and the outsiders' seem to be laughing at your situation.

The wrongs, suddenly feel normal. The abnormalities suddenly feel right. Everything you experience from that day forth, suddenly becomes frustrating to all those around you, because you feel as though your life is absolute – when it's not. You are constantly being scorned, by your family and your 'significant other.' You feel ashamed, you feel angry, and this becomes the normal, daily routine.

But what really sucks, is it feels as though you are stuck between realities. You see things differently, when knowing you died on the surgical table for a few minutes to an hour (from over hearing the staff); and suddenly, your life goes from the same ol', same ol', to, "I'm alive.

When the recovery stage, feels over, you finally go back to the job market. A financial starvation, because the 'state' wasn't there to help you, along with your community. You feel as though your life will stay in shambles, because you've been stuck in a rut for over 7 years.

You are trapping your spouse in a financial crisis, that is an ongoing storm. The bills rack up, you end up with traffic tickets you cannot pay, you fear the possibility of jail-time, or losing your drivers license, because of the penalties with not being able to pay the court. Rent is due again; you still have no money from not gaining a job.

You feel ashamed with yourself, because even a shitty job at McDonald's for just 8 hours a week, won't even hire you. Then you receive more collection notices of your monthly bills, saying that if you don't stick to a $200 payment plan for your electric, you will, get shut off; along with losing something as simple as a $45 a month internet bill, to find a job.

You finally gain employment, only to become overwhelmed with frustration and <u>hate for the job you received</u>, just to walk out of it, not realizing the harm that you just put upon yourself, and the never-ending shambles continue.

Within two weeks of being unemployed, you finally receive an over-the-phone interview, assuming you aced it. Then you receive an email, thanking you for being a good candidate, only to be, turned down. Then you tell your spouse, get into another argument, to only feel worse off than you did five minutes prior. Working up the bravery was difficult, only become scorned, once again.

Not everyone goes thru this, but I have. I cannot speak for all brain patients; only myself. I know that we all share struggles that were in relations of the type of surgery/recovery. We all seem to have gaps in our memories. We all become more frustrated with life; not knowing how we can react to a situation that we're not remembering properly. Some never recover, some do. It's sort of a 50/50 chance of recovery. There are even some that get worse, than before the surgery. The doctors are well known to nick things that can paralyze a person, even an eye –

as mine did. Depending on your state (like my own, NY), it seems as though there isn't a lawyer in the state that will sue a hospital.

For example, my friend that I had mentioned, took nearly a year of full recovery; and is back to work, and is doing exactly what he did before, just as good. I've heard of others never fully recovering; and like myself, I haven't fully recovered either. The worse thing I've experienced, that the doctor did say I'd have issues with (for the first 5, not after), is elevators. Boy, oh boy, I cannot express to you that is by far the worse thing your head can experience. It's almost as though, a shockwave enters your brain; you feel as though you could drop to your knees, and pass out - even if it's only going one floor up, or down. It's crazy, and scary, simultaneously.

In a sense, of the many surgeries people receive, there isn't many rehab programs for brain surgery patients, except for time and medication. Unless you have pins and needles on the outside, such as Tim had. Then you, are given, a rehab program for your "motor" functions. Why can they not enforce this for all brain surgery, related procedures?

I for one, after six months, had removed myself off from a medication, because I became so overweight from taking a steroid; and the doctor wouldn't replace it with something else. It cost me $4, and 80 pounds. What did they receive?

Chapter 4: SSDI, and the Courts

Living off the court system isn't as easy as one would believe. I listened to my family, by trying this route just a few years back. Nevertheless, when I listened to my family, I got denied several times. Let me notify you the quick story:

According to the courts, you must have an ongoing paper trail for your medical records. However, you cannot work, and you must keep the paper trail up. How the hell can anyone do this, while staying unemployed? Not to mention, with brain surgery, if your doctor doesn't believe you, how are you going to get them to back you, when applying for disability? How do so many people live off the system, when it doesn't give it to the people who deserve the assistance?

Here's an example.

The last time I had applied for disability insurance (SSDI), I used both my brain surgery, and my Mild Cerebral Palsy. At the time I signed up for the assistance, I had a current paper trail. I was out of work for 8 months, and by the time I had seen the judge, he said my paper work was outdated, and if I cannot get work here, I should move to another state...!

Let me get this straight. I must move out of New York, with absolutely no money – because I followed the rules of staying out of work – and they expect me to leave NY to work? In addition, the court also acted as though my Mild C.P., was suddenly a virus, or an illness, because the dipshit assumed that it could be, healed, with the proper medication or treatment (Physical Therapy). When, like the other million or so others that have Mild Cerebral Palsy (or other forms of it), cannot become cured; unless under 16 (based on an overpriced surgery). The same can be, said for people like me, who received brain surgery. But what the hell do these people know, when they've never gone thru the experience, and recovery stages that I have, or others in my position?

In my opinion, the courts aren't accepting people like me. From an appearance standpoint, I look normal – it's the story of my life. I've always appeared to be normal. My disabilities aren't posing a threat, such as a physical bias. Therefore, why should I receive assistance when from a visual standpoint, I look healthy?

Chapter 5: Being Creative

Being creative is a gift. Few have this gift, and even fewer know how to put it to good use.

I am an author. That much is obvious. I began writing books before I had my brain surgery. And something exploded within my mind thereafter the surgery.

My first book, which bombed, was "J.J.'s Rhymin' Adventures", which carried something like 25 poems of J.J. seeking adventures. Unfortunately, I didn't have pictures to go along with it, and never found the proper artist to assist.

I didn't write much after that, until a few months later, when my wife, had encouraged me to create my first novel. I laughed at the idea, because I didn't have the courage to attempt it.

A few months after my wife had brought a novel up, I had a dream, and decided to write it down. Before I realized, I was creating my first novel, "A Twist in Travel: Fate".

The novel wasn't complete when I had my brain surgery. When I came out of surgery, I had all these great, historical changing ideas. From re-writing my novel, to *flushable wipes*. Which at the time (2012), they were not, invented?

I attempted to get my cousin involved, but he thought I was nuts. It reminded me of how the idea for cell phones, "that would never work, nobody would buy such a thing". Yet, there's nearly a cellphone in every, one person's hand (including children). With the flushable wipes, they are in hospitals, schools, nurseries, homes, parents use them for their babies, adults use them to get the gunk out of their ass-cracks! They're everywhere, is my point. I could have been a multi-billionaire just from inventing flushable wipes!

That was just the first invention that I had thought of when I awoke after brain surgery. I some how managed to think of dozens of new concepts, but nobody ever took me seriously, and I'd be one of the richest people on the planet, if they had.

Since I had finished, then published both my first book, and my first novel, I have a growing collection of over the mid-50s! Just imagine, over 50 published titles on Amazon.com, since April of 2014…How many authors can say that?

With all my ideas, and my book creations, I'm still stuck in the category of *A STARVING ARTIST*. It's quite sad, really, seeming how I have much to provide for the world to learn from. I am an entrepreneur stuck in a poor-man's life. It totally sucks, I cannot express that enough. To emphasize ways of learning from me, I cannot push that upon the world enough.

I cannot tell you where these ideas are coming from. It could be the universe, God, or in some spiritual manner, that my mind & soul grabs onto from the nothingness. What I can tell you, is that the only way I will stop writing/creating books for the world, will be my demise.

Chapter 6: Which way is up?

I don't have a clue as to where I am heading. Currently, I feel lost. I'm not "depressed" in normal manners; lost I am.

Am I meant to only write/create books? Is that the only purpose I have in my shitty life? Am I the only one that sees the world in a completely different form, only to be, titled as, Crazy?

Why am I here? Is it to inspire the world with my words, my horrific theories, opinions, hypothesis, and even my fictional books? Am I supposed to stay away from the worker-bee market? Perhaps.

The one thing I am similar with other authors, is that I am stuck in my own box; even though I think outside of the box. It's a conspiracy, of how I made it this far in my life. Nearly 39 (only two weeks away; May 1), I feel as though I am searching out who I really am.

I don't know which way is up. I have been married for nearly 19 years (May 27, 2000). My wife and I have had many various ups, and downs. Thru thick and thin, sickness & and health, we've been there for one another. Nonetheless, with the way I have recovered from brain surgery, it feels as though we have grown so far apart, it's almost as though we're two different people, altogether. I hate to see her go thru such turmoil, while attempting to be the "good wife" as she stands by me, in my corner. I hate to see her feel the hellish pain of our financial crisis. Her family cannot stand that I am doing this to her, and in some aspects, I cannot blame them one bit. Nevertheless, it's clearly a brain malfunction, and something that I cannot control – except for my writing, of course. Why is it that I am only capable of committing to my writing? Am I cursed, which way is up?

Chapter 7: Am I the problem, or solution?

Am I the problem, or the solution? I cannot tell anymore. I feel as though that I am the route to all the issues in my marriage, and everything that has gone wrong in my life. This isn't self-doubt, as one could assume. This is taking a mental step back, reflecting what I have achieved, and where I should be by the time, I hit 40.

As I mentioned in the previous chapter, I will be turning 39 shortly, and I want to be damn certain that my life should be moving forward, rather than backwards – or even in a standstill.

I cannot find a "job", but I already have a career. This career has brought me to a higher level of thinking, in comparison of the normal human being living the day-to-day life, that we're all brainwashed to learn from an early age.

Why am I different? What really occurred during my brain surgery, that I have had to go thru so much change? For both good and bad…it seems to be worse than good. I'm thankful, more than you could ever know, that I am capable of creating stories, from experiences, hidden knowledge (that literally floats within my mind like an Indie car on a race track), theories (that some skeptics would refer to as conspiracy theories), hypothesis, political realism, and even fiction; such as science fiction, fantasy, thrillers, mystery, and horror.

As you may have noticed, that I jump around a lot. Both inside the material, but the types of books that I create/provide. From children's, adult fiction, driving books, losing my dog, losing my father, suicide help reference book, a biography (which must also arrange with my C.P.), and many social science-related books. I have covered many bases, and most stay true today (years after the first publication date).

Chapter 8: The first few weeks of recovery

I had a three night stay at the hospital where I had my surgery. During the day, very boring. Did you know that you must pay between $5 and $20 a day for cable in your room? Yeah, at the time I didn't.

At first, I was, of course, stoked that there was a television in my room, when I first woke. Then I found out that I'm going to be listening to all the beeping and watching a black screen from the television, along with the ongoing doctor-students checking me over from top to bottom. They should have just kept me naked, for all the checkups with my genetalia!

By the second night, the cute nurse activated the cable service for me, since I had an extremely difficult time of falling asleep. The staff was literally in my room every hour at night, to make sure I wasn't going to die. It was brutal, to say the least. Luckily, I was at least, on morphine, with codeine. The last night was the same, and they didn't cut back on the morphine, until my last hour of being in the hospital!

When I walked out of the hospital, I lit cigarette after cigarette, because there was no chance, I could sneak one, while being in the hospital. If I recall, I believe I smoked three packs that day, and I normally smoke one pack a day; sometimes almost two.

On the way home, my wife called ahead to the pharmacy to make sure the medication would be ready for pick up, and come to find out it wasn't. Those bastards made me wait three days from the time I left the hospital, before receiving any kind of medication; because my insurance didn't want to approve the type of medication. And the doctor was more than difficult to get a hold of after surgery, because he went on vacation!

Once I had received the medication, my pain vanished, as you would assume.

I wasn't supposed to take a shower for a week, so I stunk bad that first week!

When I did take my first shower, it was refreshing, followed by major disgusting. The reason, it was gross, was I had brain matter come out of my nostril, all the way down to my knees. And I'm six foot, three inches tall. Just imagine a string that comes out of your nose, that long, that you must suck back in…ewe!

I didn't have much bleeding, but the occasional speech impediment and the brain matter, it was difficult for a few months.

I recall, the first day back home, my wife took me to get a sub. I was out of it, in a ton of pain, but was hungry, and the local pizza joint was, closed at that time. Therefore, subs were about the only thing I can manage to comply with.

When my wife walked away to grab a drink (it was in a Circle K), I had to order my sub. This is what came out, ***"I would like a football, slub, on queet"***. What I meant to relay: *I would like a meatball sub, on wheat.* Big difference, right?

Things like that occurred often for the first year. My best friend became my couch, I didn't talk to many, because I hated living with a new disability. I did get my drivers license back, which was great; but I couldn't work, so it was pointless at the time. I attempted two different jobs; but neither panned out because any slight movement too fast,

made my head spin.

Chapter 9: The Conclusion

It's obvious that I've had my fair share of barriers along my journey to recovery.

I haven't gone back for my annual head-scans; because I cannot afford it, and my fear of my brain cyst returning is high. I hate doctors because of what occurred to me. All they do is guess and take my money, like they do with others. The medical environment has turned into a business, rather than a doctor, patient, relationship. You are limited one-health related issue when you visit a doctor's office. And if they don't know something, they don't take the time to find out what's wrong with you, because they'd rather just pass off medication (bandage), rather than fix the issue, or find the root to the issue.

Personally, if I had a chance to do it again, I wouldn't. If I had the chance to go back, I never would have done it, either. The doctor did inform me privately, just before surgery, that if I waited another six months, my cyst had a 97% chance of turning into a Cancerous Tumor. I almost wish I let it; but then again, I wouldn't be able to have published any books, or this one, for that matter.

When you are, dealt a shitty hand, your life feels it's trapped in Hell.

Without the right connections in life, you'll never be able to get better, with financials. They say hard work pays off. But as you can see, I'm still waiting for the results – along with my spouse.

The people I once knew, have all changed, and I don't know if my surgery is to blame, or if it's just the way I am. Give it time, and I will be all alone, and turn into a hermit.

On some aspects, it was good that I went thru the surgery; but I wasn't prepared for any of it. I think I could be better prepared for being as famous as Stephen King, then going thru Brain Surgery! Which is a humongous difference, obviously.

The moral of this book, is to inform you where your medical team hasn't. I hope this book has helped you in some way. It was difficult to create, but I am again, I wouldn't be able to have published any books, or this one, for that matter.

When you are, dealt a shitty hand, your life feels it's trapped in Hell.

Without the right connections in life, you'll never be able to get better, with financials. They say hard work pays off. But as you can see, I'm still waiting for the results – along with my spouse.

The people I once knew, have all changed, and I don't know if my surgery is to blame, or if it's just the way I am. Give it time, and I will be all alone, and turn into a hermit.

On some aspects, it was good that I went thru the surgery; but I wasn't prepared for any of it. I think I could be better prepared for being as famous as Stephen King, then going thru Brain Surgery! Which is a humongous difference, obviously.

The moral of this book, is to inform you where your medical team hasn't. I hope this book has helped you in some way. It was difficult to create, but I am glad I did; seeming how nobody really discusses this sort of thing in other books.

Please leave a review where you purchased this copy, and send me a message if you'd like to reach out; whether it's to thank me, ask me anything, or just connect. Good luck!

In addition, I would like to thank you for reading. Furthermore, not only does your old memories vanish, but you become more forgetful the longer you go after surgery. Some call it laziness, but they're ignorant for forgetting that you had brain surgery!

www.ingramcontent.com/pod-product-compliance
Lightning Source LLC
Chambersburg PA
CBHW022126170526
45157CB00004B/1779